Practical Record/ Cumulative Record

for Basic BSc (Nursing) Course

Sixth Edition

I Clement

Doctorate of Philosophy in Nursing (PhD)
MSc Nursing (Medical Surgical Nursing) MA (Sociology) MSc (Psychology)
MBA (Education) MA (Child Care and Education) MA (Education) MPhil (Education)
Postgraduate (Hospital Administration)

Presently
Professor and Head
Department of Research and Development
RV College of Nursing
Bengaluru, Karnataka, India

Formerly
Principal and Professor
Department of Medical Surgical Nursing
Columbia College of Nursing
Bengaluru, Karnataka, India

Formerly, Principal
VSS College of Nursing
Bengaluru, Karnataka, India

PhD Guide, Examiner, Thesis Evaluator
Rajiv Gandhi University of Health Sciences
Bengaluru, Karnataka, India

Chief Editor for Nursing Journals
Editorial Chief for Various International Nursing Journals

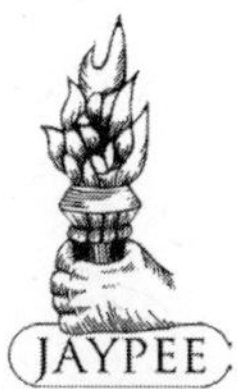

JAYPEE BROTHERS MEDICAL PUBLISHERS
The Health Sciences Publisher
New Delhi | London

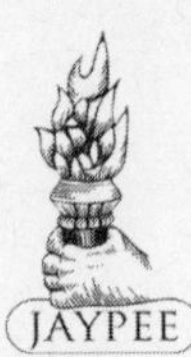

Jaypee Brothers Medical Publishers (P) Ltd.

Headquarters

Jaypee Brothers Medical Publishers (P) Ltd
EMCA House
23/23-B, Ansari Road, Daryaganj
New Delhi - 110 002, India
Landline: +91-11-23272143, +91-11-23272703
+91-11-23282021, +91-11-23245672
Email: jaypee@jaypeebrothers.com

Corporate Office

Jaypee Brothers Medical Publishers (P) Ltd
4838/24, Ansari Road, Daryaganj
New Delhi 110 002, India
Phone: +91-11-43574357
Fax: +91-11-43574314
Email: jaypee@jaypeebrothers.com

Overseas Office

J.P. Medical Ltd
83 Victoria Street, London
SW1H 0HW (UK)
Phone: +44 20 3170 8910
Fax: +44 (0)20 3008 6180
Email: info@jpmedpub.com

Website: www.jaypeebrothers.com

Website: www.jaypeedigital.com

Inquiries for bulk sales may be solicited at: jaypee@jaypeebrothers.com

Practical Record/Cumulative Record for Basic BSc (Nursing) Course

First Edition: 2008

Second Edition: 2011

Third Edition: 2012

Fourth Edition: 2016

Fifth Edition: 2018

Sixth Edition: **2022**

ISBN: 978-93-5465-238-7

Printed at: Sterling Graphics Pvt. Ltd.

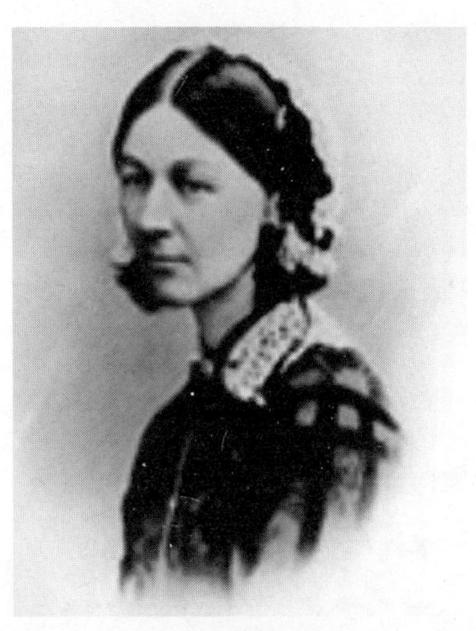

MISS FLORENCE NIGHTINGALE

PIONEER OF MODERN NURSING

Born: 12th May 1820 Died: 13th Aug 1910

Nurses Prayer

AS I CARE
FOR MY PATIENTS TODAY
BE THERE WITH ME,
OH LORD, I PRAY.
MAKE MY WORDS KIND
AND IN MY HANDS
PLACE YOUR HEALING TOUCH.
LET YOUR LOVE SHINE
THROUGH ALL THAT I DO.
SO THOSE IN NEED
MAY HEAR AND FEEL YOU.

The Nightingale Pledge

I solemnly pledge myself before God, and in the presence of this assembly, to maintain at all times, the highest standards of nursing care and to professional conduct.

I will respect the religious beliefs of patients, and will hold in confidence, all personal information entrusted to me.

I will carry out the physician's orders, intelligently and loyally, and in private life, will adhere to the standards of personal ethics, which will reflect credit upon my profession.

I will do my utmost, to fulfill the fundamental responsibility of a nurse, which is four fold: to promote health, to prevent illness, to restore health, and to alleviate suffering.

Preface to the Sixth Edition

It gives me immense pleasure to draft this sixth edition of *Practical Record/Cumulative Record for Basic BSc (Nursing) Course*. First of all I would like to thank my Lord Almighty, for His wonderful blessings who gave me strength to complete this record book in time.

Nursing is a noble service to individuals, families and society. Nursing is based on art and science that molds the attitudes, intellectual competencies and practical skills of the individual nursing student. The scope of nursing practice encompasses provision of promotive, preventive, curative and rehabilitative aspects of care to people across their lifespan in a wide variety of healthcare settings. "Practice makes a person perfect" as per this proverb, in order to practice the nursing procedures properly every nursing student requires a record book. This record book has been prepared with comprehensive approach, which will be very useful to all BSc nursing students and act as an essential tool to document their practiced skill also serve as legal evidence about their knowledge and practice as licensed nurse in future. This record book has been revised and added all required nursing procedures of nursing foundation for first year, community health nursing–I, medical surgical nursing–I in second year, medical surgical nursing–II, child health nursing, psychiatric nursing in third year, obstetric and gynecological nursing and community health nursing–II in fourth year and other subjects as recommended. Record book has been strictly prepared as per Indian Nursing Council Syllabus. It reflects initially with course distribution and highlights the required practical hours, for respective subjects gives idea about setting a target to complete the procedures, as per requirement it also has the separate allocation to get documented after being supervised and students can get signed for demonstration and re-demonstration of nursing procedure and other required practical procedures for completion of the course. Definitely this record book will help all the students to practice a comprehensive approach to integrate theory into practice.

I am sure that all students will use this book to practice the nursing procedures.

I Clement

Preface to the First Edition

Nursing procedures are the vital components in a clinical practice, which requires thorough knowledge and adequate and repeated practices. These procedures should be learnt in an organized fashion by using excellent practical record, which needs to fulfill the requirements of Indian Nursing Council and Rajiv Gandhi University of Health Sciences, Bengaluru, Karnataka, India.

The nursing procedures may be demonstrated at the classrooms, laboratories, and wards by the nursing tutors/clinical instructors/ward incharges. The nursing students are expected to pay attention, take up initiation and interest to do active participation to learn the new skills. Nursing procedures are life-oriented procedures, so the human concerns, values and ethical components should be taken into consideration.

The record would provide the information regarding the practical experience gained by the student nurse under strict clinical supervision during the course. The procedures carried out or learned by the student in all the specialties, according to year-wise, are listed out. This procedure record is a written document, which is very important for the students as well as for the teacher to assist the learning process of the student and it is a clinical evidence.

The nursing students take opportunity to practice the procedure in the clinical areas as early as possible. When the student nurse is efficient in his/her skill and knowledge of a particular procedure, signature should be obtained from the clinical instructor/supervisor in the columns provided.

The nursing procedure should be learnt by using the scientific principles of nursing such as uniformity, simple to complex and to save time, money, material and energy. The practical record should be certified by the class-coordinator and the principal every year before the annual practical examination and should be submitted to the examiners at the time of board examination.

I Clement

Guidelines to Use the Practical Record

General Objectives

Students will be able to understand, comprehend, correlate the theory with practice and develop skills in performing various procedures based on scientific principles and rationale for every step adapted.

Contributory Objectives

In the clinical posting, students will be able to:

1. Correlate the theory with practice.
2. Practice the learnt scientific principles for each procedure done for the patient.
3. Assemble all the articles required for the procedure.
4. Demonstrate the skills in performing the procedure accurately.
5. Develop and apply the skills in assessment, planning, implementation with rationale and evaluating the nursing care in hospital and in community.
6. Perform the steps of any procedure systematically and provide care based on priority needs of patient.
7. Assess the learning needs of patient and provide health education.
8. Develop ability to record and report.

Instruction for Proper Use of Procedure Record/Cumulative Record

1. Procedure record is a clinical evidence of each student; therefore, every student needs to handle this record carefully, keep it safe, and fulfill requirements mentioned in the record.
2. Procedure record front page regarding student's information to be filled, fix passport size photograph, cover the record and label it.
3. Procedure once demonstrated with the theory in the laboratory (or) in class, students are expected to do re-demonstration under supervision of nursing staff, signatures to be given in demonstration column with the date by the respective staff after conducting viva about the procedure done.
4. Procedure done by the student in the clinical should get signature in the clinical column after performing three times, to ensure satisfaction by the staff after attending viva of the same procedure.
5. Rough signature for the same procedure to be obtained in the rough book, after completing three rough signatures, a fair signature is done in the cumulative record with date and time.
6. Students who put duplicate signature will be severely punished (or) will undergo strict disciplinary action.
7. Students are not allowed to overwrite (or) do any writing (or) scrabble anything in the procedure book.
8. Students are expected to complete the procedure for each year, two weeks prior to university examination, get signature and submit to principal, those who fail to complete procedure book will be not eligible for the university examination and practical.
9. Students who lost this cumulative record are responsible for themselves, should get signatures completely in a new record at their own risk to their respective teachers by showing rough signatures obtained previously in the rough practical book.
10. No student is permitted to do any procedure independently unless she/he obtained signature for that procedure under supervision.
11. Student is expected to take responsibility for her/his own learning by:
    a. Requesting the clinical instructors to supervise the procedure she/he needs to have signature.
    b. Volunteering for experience she/he needs.
    c. Taking responsibility for obtaining signature from the clinical instructor who supervised the procedure, immediately following successful completion of procedure and attending viva regarding the same.
12. Student should ensure that they get signature from internal and external examiners after successful completion of practical examination each year.
13. Students who have back up in their academic activities, should get signature in the area from internal and external examiners, after completing their practical examination.
14. Staff should not delay (or) hesitate to give signature in time, ensure all the procedures done are signed properly with date.

Clinical Experience Record

Name of the Institution: ______________________________

____

Name of the Student: ______________________________
(In BLOCK LETTERS)

____

Registration No: ______________________________

Passport size photo

Age and Date of Birth: ______________________________

Father's Name: ______________________________

Date of Joining the Course: ______________________________

Date of Completion: ______________________________

Permanent Address: ______________________________

____

Signature of the Student

Date:

Signature of the Principal

Date:

College Seal

Contents

First Year

- Hours of Instruction 1
- Distribution of Subjects and Marks 2
- Nursing Foundations 3
- Nutrition Practicals 12
- Practical Examination 14
- Nursing Foundation–Evaluation Performa 15

Second Year

- Hours of Instruction 16
- Distribution of Subjects and Marks 17
- Medical Surgical Nursing-I 18
- Community Health Nursing-I 26
- Communication and Educational Technology 28
- Clinical Evaluation 30
- Practical Examination 32

Third Year

- Hours of Instruction 33
- Distribution of Subjects and Marks 33
- Medical Surgical Nursing-II 34
- Child Health Nursing 40
- Mental Health Nursing 45
- Practical Examination 49
- Clinical Evaluation 50

Fourth Year

- Hours of Instruction 52
- Distribution of Subjects and Marks 52
- Midwifery and Obstetrical Nursing (Normal) 53
- Midwifery and Obstetrical Nursing (Abnormal) 57
- Community Health Nursing-II 61
- Clinical Evaluation for Community Health Nursing-II 65
- Nursing Administration 66
- Practical Examination 67
- Nursing Research and Statistics 68
- Clinical Posting 69

First Year

FIRST YEAR
HOURS OF INSTRUCTION

Theory: 930 hours **Clinical Experiences: 450 hours**

Sl. No.	*Subjects*	*Theory (Hours)*	*Practical (Hours)*	
1.	English	60		
2.	Regional Language	30	-	
3.	Anatomy	60	-	
4.	Physiology	60	-	
5.	Nutrition	60	-	
6.	Biochemistry	30	-	
7.	Nursing Foundation	465	450	
8.	Psychology	60	-	
9.	Microbiology	60	-	
10.	Introduction to Computers	45	-	
11.	Library Work/Self-Study	-	-	50
12.	Co-curricular Activities	-	-	50
	Total	**930**	**450**	**100**
	Total Number of Hours: 1480			

Distribution of Subjects and Marks for Internal Assessment and University Examination

Sl. No.	*Subjects*	*Hours*	*Internal assessment*	*External assessment*	*Total*
1.	Anatomy and Physiology	3	25	75	100
2.	Nutrition and Biochemistry	3	25	75	100
3.	Nursing Foundation	3	25	75	100
4.	Psychology	3	25	75	100
5.	Microbiology	3	25	75	100
6.	English	2		50	50
7.	Introduction to Computer	2		50	50
	Practical and Viva				
	Nursing Foundation		**100**	**100**	**200**

Note: Introduction to Computer and English as college examination, respective college will conduct examination and marks to be sent to the university.

Attendance of the student (%) :

Theory :

Clinical :

Signature of Class Coordinator *Signature of the Principal*

FIRST YEAR
NURSING FOUNDATIONS

Sl. No.	Subjects	Demonstration in foundation lab		Clinical	
		Date	Signature	Date	Signature
1.	**Hospital Admission**				
	Admission				
	Prepare unit for new patient				
	Prepare admission bed				
	Perform admission procedure				
	Emergency admission				
	Routine admission				
	Transfer in				
	Prepare patient records				
2.	**Hospital Discharge**				
	Discharge counseling				
	Perform discharge procedure				
	Planned discharge				
	Leave against medical advice (LAMA)/ Discharge against medical advice (DAMA)				
	Absconded				
	Referrals and transfer out				
	Medico legal case (MLC) cases				
	Prepare patient records				
	Disinfect the units				
	Disinfect the equipment				
3.	**Nursing Process**				
	History taking				
	Nursing assessment				
	Physical examination				
	Nursing diagnosis				
	Problem list				
	Prioritization				
	Outcome/goals				
	Selection intervention				
	Nursing Process Application				
	Writing nursing care plan				
4.	**Communication**				
	Verbal techniques				
	Nonverbal techniques				
	Interpersonal communication				
	Therapeutic communication				
	Patient teaching sessions				
	Maintaining Communication with Patient and Family				

Contd...

Contd...

5.	**Recording and Reporting**				
	Change of shift reports				
	Transfer reports				
	Incident reports				
	Patient report presentation				
	Documentation & Reporting				
	Documentation of Patient care and Procedures				
	Verbal Report				
	Written Report				
6.	**Vital Signs**				
	Temperature				
	• Oral				
	• Axillary				
	• Tympanic				
	• Rectal				
	Pulse				
	Apical pulse				
	Peripheral pulse				
	Respiration				
	Blood pressure				
	Recording vital signs				
	Recording vital sign in graphical sheet				
	Pulse oxymetry				
	Pain assessment by using pain scale				
7.	**Health Assessment**				
	Health history taking				
	Perform assessment				
	General assessment body system				
	Methods of physical exam				
	• Head to toe examination				
	• System vice examination				
	Inspection				
	Palpation				
	Percussion				
	Auscultation				
	Olfaction				
	Identification of system vice deviation				
	Documentation of findings				
8.	**Patients Unit Preparations**				
	Bed making				
	Prepare beds				
	Open bed				

Contd...

Contd...

	Closed bed				
	Occupied bed				
	Operation bed				
	Amputation bed				
	Cardiac bed				
	Fracture bed				
	Burns bed				
	Divided bed				
	Fowler's bed				
	Pain assessment and provision of comfort				
9.	**Comfort Devices**				
	Extra pillows				
	Back rest				
	Cardiac table				
	Sand bag				
	Bed cradle				
	Trochanter rolls				
	Cotton ring and hand rolls				
	Air cushion				
	Water and air mattress				
	Foot end elevator				
	Air mattress				
	Water mattress				
10.	**Safety Devices/Care**				
	Restraints (Physical)				
	Protective padding				
	Side rails				
	Care of pressure points				
	Fall Risk Assessment				
	Post Fall Assessment				
11.	**Hygienic Needs**				
	Oral hygiene				
	Morning and evening care				
	Bed bath				
	• Partial bath				
	• Sponge bath				
	Assisted bed bath				
	Care of Skin				
	Back care				
	• Back massage				
	• Care of pressure points				
	• Pressure sore risk assessment—Norton Scale				

Contd...

Contd...

	Hair care				
	Bed shampoo or hair wash				
	Pediculosis treatment				
	Care of hand and feet				
	Perineal care				
12.	**Nutritional Needs**				
	Nutritional assessment				
	Preparation of nasogastic tube food				
	Nasogastric tube insertion				
	Nasogstric tube conformation				
	Nasogastric tube feeding				
	Gastrostomy feeding				
	Parenteral feeding				
	Nasogastric suction/aspiration				
	Nasogastric irrigation				
13.	**Urinary Elimination**				
	Provides urinals/bedpan				
	Condom drainage				
	Perineal care				
	Catheterization				
	• Male				
	• Female				
	Urinary catheter care				
	Care of urinary drainage				
	Bladder irrigation				
	Maintaining urinary output chart				
	Findenting urinary problems				
14.	**Bowel Elimination**				
	Assessment of bowel				
	Determining bowel sounds				
	Provides bedpan				
	Insertion of flatus tube				
	Enema				
	Insertion of suppository				
	Bowel wash				
	Identifying bowel problems				
	• Diarrhea				
	• Constipation				
15.	**Mobility and Exercise**				
	Mobility assessment				
	Range of motion exercises				
	Changing position of helpless patient				
	Transfer from bed to wheel chair, trolley				
	Ambulation				

Contd...

Contd...

16.	**Positions**				
	Recumbent				
	Lateral (Right/Left)				
	Fowlers				
	Sim's				
	Lithotomy				
	Prone				
	Trendelenburg				
	Knee chest				
	Maintaining position chart				
17.	**Oxygen Administration**				
	Assessment of oxygen status				
	Simple face mask				
	Nasal cannula				
	Venture mask				
	Oxyhood				
	Oropharyngeal				
	Nasopharyngeal				
	Care of oxygen cylinder				
	Pulse oximeter monitoring				
	Identifying Hypoxic condition				
18.	**Therapeutic Procedures**				
	Chest physiotherapy				
	Postural drainage				
	Care of chest drainage				
	CPR-Basic				
	Intravenous therapy				
	Blood transfusions				
	Blood and blood component therapy				
	Identifications of side effects				
	Documentation of therapeutic procedures				
19.	**Specimen Collection**				
	Urine: routine, culture and 24 hours				
	Stool: routine and culture				
	Blood: routine, culture				
	Peripheral blood smear				
	Sugar: strip/glucometer, GRBS monitoring				
	Vomitus				
	Throat swab				
	Urine test: reaction, specific gravity, albumin and sugar				

Contd...

Contd...

	Documentation specimen collection				
	Transport of specimen to the laboratory				
20.	**Hot Applications**				
	Hot water bag				
	Hot fomentation				
	Steam inhalation				
	Sitz bath				
	Hot packs				
	Interpret and report alterations				
21.	**Cold Applications**				
	Cold compress				
	Ice cap				
	Tepid sponge				
	Cold sponging				
	Use of cold drinks				
	Interpret and report alterations				
22.	**Care of Specially Disabled and Common Illness**				
	Assessment of specially disabled				
	Visually impaired				
	Hearing impaired				
	Mentally challenged				
	Care of patient with fever				
	Care of patient with dyspnea				
	Care patient with cast and traction				
	Care of patient with diarrhea				
	Care of patient with paralysis				
	Care of patient with constipation				
	Care of patient with urinary retention				
	Care of patient with incontinence				
	Care of patient with vomiting/anorexia				
	Care of patient with acute and chronic pain				
	Care of patient with unconsciousness				
	Glasgow coma scale				
23.	**Infection Control**				
	Hand washing techniques				
	• Medical hand washing				
	• Surgical hand washing—Scrub				
	Preparation of isolation unit				
	Practice techniques of wearing and removing personal protective equipment				
	Disposal of waste				

Contd...

Contd...

	Infection control measures				
	Social distancing				
	Wearing mask				
	Gloving technique				
	Growing technique				
24.	**Universal Precautions**				
	Personal protective equipment (PPE)				
	Surgical wears				
	• Mask				
	• Gown				
	• Gloves				
	• Cap				
	• Aprons				
	• Shoes				
	• Goggles				
	Social isolation				
	Barrier technique				
	Reverse barrier technique				
	Respiratory isolation				
25.	**Decontamination of Equipment and Unit**				
	Surgical asepsis				
	Medical asepsis				
	Sterilization				
	Handling sterilized equipment				
	Calculate strengths of lotions				
	Prepare lotions				
	Care of articles				
	Fumigation				
	Terminal sterilization				
26.	**Pre- and Postoperative Care**				
	Pre- and Post-operative assessment				
	Skin preparation for surgery				
	Preparation of postoperative unit preparation				
	Pre- and postoperative teaching and counseling				
	Preoperative preparation				
	• Physical				
	• Psychological				
	• Physiological				
	• Informed consent				
	• Pharmacological				
	• Spiritual				

Contd...

Contd...

	Pre- and postoperative monitoring				
	Care of wound				
	Surgical care				
	Suture care				
	Care of drainage				
	Documentation in pre- and postoperative care				
	Identification of complication				
27.	**Medication Administration**				
	Principles of medication administration				
	Rights of medication administration				
	Administration of medications in different forms and routes				
	Oral, sublingual and buccal				
	Intradermal				
	Subcutaneous				
	Intramuscular				
	Assist with intravenous medications				
	Drug measurements and dose calculation				
	Preparations of lotions and solutions				
	Administers topical applications				
	Insertion of drug into body cavity				
	• Suppository				
	• Medicated packs				
	Instillation of medications and sprays				
	• Ear				
	• Nose				
	• Eyes				
	• Throat				
	• Bladder				
	• Vagina				
	• Rectum				
	Inhalation: moist and dry				
	Documentation in medication administration				
	Medication error				
28.	**First Aid and Bandaging**				
	Principles of first aid				
	Priorities in first aid				
	• Preparation of first aid kit				
	• Snake bite				
	• Accident/bleeding				
	• Shock				

Contd...

Contd...

	• Burns				
	• Epistaxis				
	• Foreign body: Eye, ear, nose and throat				
	• Fracture				
	• Poisoning				
	• Other emergencies				
	CPR-Code blue, crash cort, procedure				
	Documentation in first aid				
	Bandaging				
	• Simple spiral				
	• Reverse spiral				
	• Figure of eight				
	• Head/capline				
	• Eyes, ear, jaw, finger, elbow and knee				
	• Use of triangular bandages				
	• Use of slings				
	• Use of binders				
	Spica				
	a. Thumb				
	b. Shoulder				
29.	**Care of Death and Dying**				
	Care of dying patient				
	Caring and packing of dead body				
	Counseling and supporting of grieving relatives				
	Terminal care of the unit				
	Hospice care				
	Palliative care				
	Care of dead bodies of infectious diseases				
	Protocol for disposal of dead bodies				
	Headling dead bodies in MLC Cases				
	Postpartum				
	Autopsy				
30.	**Observational Visit and Write Report**				
	Health agency				
	CFTRI				
	Milk diary				
	CSSD and infection control unit				
	Clinical pathology and biochemistry lab				
	Blood bank				
	Hospital visit				

NUTRITION PRACTICALS

Sl. No.	*Nursing Procedures*	*Date of demo in lab*	*Supervisors signature*
1.	**Nutritional Assessment**		
2.	**Preservation and Storage of foods**		
3.	**Preparation of**		
	Balanced diet		
	Weaning diet		
	Family diet and menu planning		
4.	**Therapeutic diet or modified diet**		
	High protein diet		
	High caloric diet		
	Salt restricted diet		
	Low fat diet		
	Diabetic diet		
	Fiber diet		
5.	**Diet planning for**		
	Pregnant mother		
	Lactating mother		
6.	**Liquid/fluid diet**		
	Tea/coffee		
	Fruit juice		
	Barley water		
	Albumin water		
	Lime juice		
	Egg flip		
	Lassi		
	Dhal soup		
	Vegetable soup		
	Meat soup		
	Bone soup		
	Milk soup		
	Butter milk		
	Orange juice		
	Tomato juice and soup		
	Grape juice		
7.	**Light diet**		
	Toast		
	Porridge		
	Salade		
	Jelly		
	Arrowroot		
	Boiled egg		
	Steamed fish		

Contd...

Contd...

	Omelette		
	Gruel		
	Kanji		
8.	**Carbohydrate**		
	Rice kheer		
	Kichidi		
	Rawa porridge		
	Ragi porridge		
	Rawa upma		
	Banana milk shake		
9.	**Proteins**		
	Sprouted grams		
	Milk and egg preparations		
	Ground nut milk shake		
	Boiled eggs		
10.	**High proteins**		
	Steamed fish		
	Steamed meat		
	Meat curry		
	Dhal preparations		
	Vada		
11.	**Diet in disease**		
	Diabetic diet		
	Cardiac diet		
	Renal diet		
	Hypertensive diet		
	Naturopathic diet		
	Diet for gout patients		
	Diet for fever patients		
	Diet for peptic ulcer patients		
	Diet for antenatal women		
	Diet for lactating mother		

Class Coordinator *Principal*

Nursing Care Plan

Sl. No.	*Care Plan*	*Date*	*Signature*
1.			
2.			
3.			
4.			
5.			

Demonstration of Physical Examination

Sl. No.		Date	Signature
1.			
2.			

Case Presentation/Ward Teaching

Sl. No.		Date	Signature
1.			
2.			
3.			
4.			

Health Education

Date	Topic	AV-Aids	Place	Individual/group	Signature
1.					
2.					

Signature of Class Coordinator *Signature of the Principal*

PRACTICAL EXAMINATION

Nursing Foundations Practical

Signature of Internal Examiner *Signature of External Examiner*

Date:

Repeat:

Signature of Internal Examiner *Signature of External Examiner*

Date:

Repeat:

Signature of Internal Examiner *Signature of External Examiner*

Date:

BSc NURSING CLINICAL EXPERIENCES–EVALUATION PERFORMA FOR NURSING FOUNDATION–PRACTICALS

Name: Ward:

Date: Total Marks: 25×4 = 100

KEY: 1. Unsatisfactory; 2. Satisfactory; 3. Good; 4. Very Good

Sl. No.		*1*	*2*	*3*	*4*
1.	Taking nursing history				
	Makes observations of patients condition				
	Identifies the basic health needs/problems				
	Priorities the needs/problems				
2.	**Planning**				
	Plans nursing care on the basis of priority				
	Plans care according to patients psychosocial needs				
	Involves patients and family in planning				
	Plans health teaching for patients				
3.	**Implementation**				
	Carries out plans based on priorities				
	Integrates scientific principles in giving care				
	Uses technical skill				
	Maintains accuracy in care				
	Controls the environment to provide for safety				
	Demonstrates initiative in implementing nursing care				
	Records significantly information to appropriate personnel				
	Communicates significant information to appropriate personnel				
	Instructs the patient and family related to their learning needs				
4.	**Evaluation**				
	Evaluates with guidance the care given				
	Modifies the plan as indicated in the evaluation				
5.	**Professional Behavior**				
	Grooming				
	Punctuality				
	Dependability				
	Interpersonal relations				
	Emotional stability				
	Professional and personal growth				
	Total				

Clinical Instructor Signature

Date:

Signature of the Student *Signature of the HOD* *Signature of the Principal*

Second Year

SECOND YEAR
HOURS OF INSTRUCTION

Theory: 510 hours **Clinical Experiences: 885 hours**

Sl. No.	*Subjects*	*Theory (Hours)*	*Practical (Hours)*	
1.	Sociology	60	-	
2.	Pharmacology	45	-	
3.	Pathology	30	-	
4.	Genetics	15	-	
5.	Medical Surgical Nursing (Adult Including Geriatrics)	210	720	
6.	Community Health Nursing	90	135	
7.	Communication and Educational Technology	60	30	
8.	Library Work/Self-Study	-	-	50
9.	Co-curricular Activities	-	-	35
	Total	**510**	**885**	**85**
	TOTAL HOURS: 1480			

Distribution of Subjects and Marks for Internal Assessment and University Examination

Sl. No.	*Subjects*	*Hours*	*Internal assessment*	*External assessment*	*Total*
1.	Sociology	3	25	75	100
2.	Medical Surgical Nursing-I	3	25	75	100
3.	Pharmacology, Pathology and Genetics	3	25	75	100
4.	Community Health Nursing-I	3	25	75	100
5.	Communication and Educational Technology	3	25	75	100
	Practical and Viva Voce				
1.	**Medical Surgical Nursing-I**		**100**	**100**	**200**

Attendance of the student (%) :

Theory :

Clinical :

Signature of Class Coordinator

Signature of the Principal

SECOND YEAR
MEDICAL SURGICAL NURSING-I

Sl. No.	*Subjects*	*Demonstration in medical surgical nursing lab*		*Clinical*	
		Date	*Signature*	*Date*	*Signature*
1.	**Nursing Care of Adult Patient with Medical Disorders**				
	Assessment of patient				
	History taking				
	Perform general and specific physical examination				
	Identify the alterations and deviations				
	Practice medical surgical safety measure				
	Standard safety measures				
	Counseling and education				
	Documentation of assessment findings				
2.	**Medication Administration**				
	Oral, sublingual, buccal				
	Intradermal				
	Subcutaneous				
	Intramuscular				
	Intravenous				
	Intravenous therapy				
	Intravenous calculation				
	Maintenance and monitoring				
	Administration of IV medications				
	Care of patient with central lines				
	Medication administration by infusion pumps				
	Documentation in medication administration				
3.	**Therapeutic Procedures**				
	Oxygen therapy—different methods				
	Nebulization				
	Chest-physiotherapy				
	Nasogastric feeding				
	Blood and component therapy				
	Throat suctioning				
	Maintain elimination				
	Catheterization				
	Bladder irrigation				
	Bowel wash				
	Enema				
	Colostomy irrigation and care				
	Urinary elimination				
	Maintain intake output chart				

Contd...

Contd...

	Hemodialysis				
	Peritoneal dialysis				
	Care of AV Shunt tubes				
	Identification of abnormal conditions				
	Documentation of procedure				
4.	**Diagnostic Procedures**				
	Invasive and non-invasive tests				
	Electrocardiogram				
	Doppler studies				
	Central venous pressure				
	Abdominal paracentesis				
	Lumbar puncture				
	Gastric lavage				
	Sternal puncture				
	Thoracocentesis				
	Cystoscopy				
	Cystometrogram				
	Intravenous pyelogram and kidney, ureter, bladder (KUB)				
	Barium enema				
	Renal biopsy				
	Liver biopsy				
	Protoscopy				
	Endoscopy				
	Cholecystography				
	Esophagogastroduodenoscopy				
	Blood studies				
	Thyroid function test				
	FBS/ PPBS/ RBS				
	Glucose tolerance test				
	Liver function test				
	Pulmonary function test				
	Interpretation of various tests				
	Identification of abnormal results				
	Documentation of diagnostic tests				
5.	**Pre- and Postoperative Nursing Care**				
	Preoperative nursing				
	• Skin preparation: local and general surgery				
	• Physiological preparation				
	• Psychological preparation				
	• Informed consent				
	• Spiritual preparation				
	• Pharmacological preparations (pre-medications)				

Contd...

Contd...

	• Preoperative checklist				
	• Teaching preoperative exercises				
	• Documentation in preoperative care				
	Postoperative nursing				
	• Setting up postoperative unit				
	• Postoperative assessment				
	• Pain: assessment and management				
	• Postoperative care: immediate and late care				
	• Recovery room care				
	• Care of wound and drainage				
	• Suture removal				
	• Surgical sock				
	• Sitz bath				
	• Ambulation and exercise				
	• Nasogastric aspiration				
	• Care of chest drainage				
	• Ostomy care: gastrostomy and colostomy				
	• Blood and component therapy				
	• Practice universal precautions				
	• Postoperative exercises				
	• Maintenance of ICU flowchart				
	• Identification of alterations				
	• Documentation of postoperative care				
6.	**Nursing Care of Adult Patient with Cardiac Disorders**				
	Cardiac assessment				
	Physical examination				
	Cardiac monitoring				
	Electrocardiogram				
	Assisting diagnostic procedures				
	Non-invasive				
	• Electrocardiogram				
	• Stress ECG				
	• Echocardiogram				
	• Radiological investigations: X-ray, computed tomography (CT), magnetic resonance imaging (MRI), positron emission tomography (PET)				
	• Recording and interpreting ECG				
	Invasive				
	• Cardiac catheterization				
	• Cardiac enzymes				
	• Central venous pressure				
	• Pulmonary artery wedge pressure				
	• Arterial blood gas analysis: Interpretations				
	• Blood sample for cardiac studies				
	Administer cardiac drugs				

Contd...

Contd...

	Assisting therapeutic procedures				
	• Percutaneous transluminal coronary angioplasty				
	• Thrombolytic therapy				
	Cardiopulmonary resuscitation				
	Cardiac rehabilitation				
	Teach patients and families				
	Practice medical and surgical asepsis				
	Standard safety measures				
	Application of anti-embolism stockings (TED hose)				
	Application/maintenance of sequential compression device				
	Identification of alterations				
	Documentation of cardiac conditions				
7.	**Intensive Care Nursing**				
	Intensive care assessment				
	Setting up of emergency trolley				
	Cardiac monitoring				
	Pulse oximeter monitoring				
	Suctioning				
	• Oropharyngeal				
	• Endotracheal				
	• Tracheostomy				
	Assisting				
	• Endotracheal intubation				
	• Ventilator care				
	• Defibrillation				
	Administration drug through infusion pump				
	Emergency drugs				
	Maintain ICU Flowchart				
	Documentation in ICU				
8.	**Nursing Care of Adult Patient with Skin Disorders**				
	Assessment of patient				
	Physical examination				
	Assisting diagnostic procedures: invasive and non-invasive				
	Assisting therapeutic procedures				
	Administration of topical medications				
	Intra-dermal injection-skin allergy testing				
	Skin biopsy				
	Blood examination for dermatological conditions				
	Practice medical surgical asepsis				
	Standard safety measures				
	Use of personal protective equipment				

Contd...

Contd...

	Providing medicated bath				
	Identification of alterations				
	Documentation of dermatological conditions				
9.	**Nursing Care of Adult Patient with Skeletomuscular Disorders**				
	Skeletomuscular assessment				
	Physical examination				
	Non-invasive procedures				
	• Radiological: X-ray, CT and MRI				
	• Muscle: tone and strength				
	Invasive				
	• Blood examination				
	• Bone marrow studies				
	• Bone biopsy				
	• Myelogram				
	Assist in application and removal of plaster cast				
	Application of traction				
	• Skin traction				
	• Skeletal traction				
	• Bucks extension traction				
	Assist in application and removal of prosthesis				
	Care of orthotics				
	Muscle strengthening exercises				
	Crutch walking				
	Rehabilitation				
	Physiotherapy				
	• Range of motion exercises				
	• Muscle strengthen exercises				
	• Crutch maneuvering technique				
	Activities of daily living				
	Ambulation				
	Teach and counsel patients and families				
	Stump care				
	Documentation in skeletomuscular conditions				
10.	**Communicable diseases**				
	Assessment in infectious Diseases				
	Physical examination				
	Diagnosis infectious diseases: invasive and non-invasive				
	• Blood examination				
	• Nasal swab				
	• Sputum collection				
	• Cervical Swab				

Contd...

Contd...

	Universal precaution				
	Isolation techniques				
	Reverse barrier nursing				
	Standard precautions				
	Handling PPE Kit				
	Needle and sharp injury prevention				
	Cleaning and disinfection				
	Respiratory hygiene				
	Waste disposal				
	Safe injection practices				
	Pandemic guidelines and procedures				
	Control measures of epidemic and pandemic outbreaks				
	Safety measures: patient and staff				
	Documentation of infectious conditions				
11.	**Operation Theater Nursing**				
	Packing of articles for surgery				
	Surgical scrubbing				
	Gowning and gloving				
	Identify instruments used for common surgeries				
	Identify suturing materials used for common surgeries				
	Disinfection of OT				
	• Carbolization				
	• Fumigation				
	Preparation of instrument sets for common operations				
	Setting up of sterile trolley for surgery				
	Sterilization of sharp and other instruments				
	Preparing the OT table depending upon the operation				
	Positioning and draping for surgery				
	Assisting in anesthesia				
	Monitoring the patient				
	Endotracheal intubation				
	Handling specimens				
	Disposal of waste as per the guidelines				
	Intraoperative monitoring				
	Assisting in major and minor operations				
	Assisting in major surgeries				
	1.				
	2.				
	3.				
	4.				
	5.				

Contd...

	Assisting in minor surgeries				
	1.				
	2.				
	3.				
	4.				
	5.				
	Equipment used in OT				
	Monitoring the patient during surgery				
	Documentation in intraoperative care				
12.	**Observational Visit**				
	Blood bank and participation in blood camps				
	Orientation visit to hospital control system				

Nursing Care Plan

Sl. No.	*Care plan*	*Date*	*Signature*
1.			
2.			
3.			
4.			
5.			

Case Studies

Sl. No.		*Date*	*Signature*
1.			
2.			
3.			
4.			

Case Presentation / Ward Teaching

Sl. No.		*Date*	*Signature*
1.			
2.			
3.			
4.			

Health Education: Individual/Group OPD/Ward

Sl. No.	*Topic*	*Date*	*Signature*
1.			
2.			
3.			
4.			

Internship-Medical Surgical Nursing-I: 260 Hours–9 Weeks

Sl. No.		Date	Signature
1.	**ICU/CCU/Cardiac OT**		
	Perform arterial puncture-5		
	Read and take ECG-5		
	Tracheostomy suctioning-5		
	Oxygen administration by CPAP mask		
	Use AMBU bag		
	Conduct and analysis of pulse oximeter		
	Assist in endotracheal intubation		
	Setting up of ventilator		
	Maintain drug sheet		
	Care of patient in ventilator		
2.	**Neuro–ICU/ITU/OT**		
	Assess the neurological status		
	Maintain drug sheet		
	Pre- and postoperative care of patient undergone neurosurgery		
3.	**Burns Unit**		
	Assessment of severity of burns		
	Care of patient with burns		
	Administer rehydration therapy		
	Observe reconstructive surgery		
	OT-Laparoscopic/orthopedic/eye/ENT		
	Identify instruments		
	Assist in OT-5 cases		
	Completed Internship requirements (260 hours)-9 weeks		

Signature of Class Coordinator *Signature of the Principal*

SECOND YEAR
COMMUNITY HEALTH NURSING-I

Sl. No.	*Subjects*	*Community lab*		*Clinical*	
		Date	*Signature*	*Date*	*Signature*
1.	**Identification of Health Determinants of Community**				
2.	**Conduct Community Survey**				
3.	**Conduct Family Health Survey**				
4.	**Report Presentation on Survey**				
5.	**Techniques of IPR**				
6.	**Family Care**				
	• History taking				
	• Physical examination				
7.	**Demonstrate Bag Technique**				
8.	**Community Nursing Procedures**				
	• Hand washing				
	• Recording vital signs				
	• Urine: sugar and albumin				
	• Nutritional assessment				
	• Hemoglobin analysis				
	• Wound dressing				
9.	**Comprehensive Family Nursing Care—Urban**				
10.	**Comprehensive Family Nursing Care—Rural**				
11.	**Collection of Specimen**				
	• Urine				
	• Sputum				
	• Blood smear				
	• Thick smear				
	• Thin smear				
12.	**Preparation of Audio-visual Aids**				
	• Flannel graph				
	• Flash cards				
	• Flip charts				
	• Posters				
	• Bulletin boards				
	• Puppet show				
13.	**Health Education**				
	• Individual				
	• Group				
	• Community-mass				

Contd...

Contd...

14.	**Participate in Family Welfare Program**				
	• Oral contraceptives				
	• Injectable contraceptives				
	• Condoms—male and female				
	• Assisting in copper-T-insertion				
	• Assisting in permanent method of sterilization				
	• Assisting in MTP/abortions				
15.	**Participate in PHC Clinics**				
16.	**Participate in Immunization Program**				
17.	**Observational Visits**				
	• Primary health center				
	• Sub-center				
	• Community health center				
	• Anganwadi				
	• Postpartum center				
	• Sewage treatment plant				
	• Water purification center				
	• Slaughter house				
	• Family planning association of India				
	• Anganwadis program				

Family Studies

Sl. No.	*Name of the head of the family*	*Identified health problems*	*Duration of study*	*Signature*
1.				
2.				
3.				
4.				
5.				

Health Teaching

Sl. No.	*Topic*	*Focused group*	*AV-Aids*	*Method*	*Date*	*Signature*
1.						
2.						
3.						
4.						
5.						

Signature of Class Coordinator *Signature of the Principal*

SECOND YEAR
COMMUNICATION AND EDUCATIONAL TECHNOLOGY

Total Hours Practical: 30 hours

Sl. No.	Subjects	Classroom		Clinical	
		Date	Signature	Date	Signature
1.	**Preparation of Rotation Plan**				
	Individual rotation plan				
	Master rotation plan				
	Clinical rotation plan				
2.	**Preparation of**				
	Unit plan				
	Course plan				
	Lesson plan				
3.	**Guidance and Counseling**				
	Organization of counseling services				
	• Individual				
	• Group				
	Managing disciplinary problems				
4.	**Method Used in Teaching Practices**				
	Classroom method:				
	• Lecture method				
	• Demonstration method				
	• Discussion method				
	• Seminar presentation				
	• Project method				
	• Symposium				
	Clinical methods:				
	• Nursing clinics				
	• Nursing rounds				
	• Nursing conference				
	• Process recording				
	• Field trips				
5.	**Preparation of Teaching Aids**				
	Nonprojected aids:				
	• Charts				
	• Chalk board				
	• Posters				
	• Flash cards				
	Projected aids:				
	• Transparencies				
	• LCD				

Contd...

Contd...

	Three dimensional aids:				
	• Models				
	• Puppets				
	Printed aids:				
	• Pamphlets				
	• Leaflets				
6.	**Preparation of Evaluation Tools**				
	Classroom tools:				
	• Objective type				
	• Subjective type				
	Clinical tools:				
	• Checklist				
	• Rating scale				
	• Observational				
	• Interview				
	• Anecdotal				
7.	**Observational Visits to School/College of Nursing and Presentation of Reports**				
	a. Libraries				
	b. College of Nursing				
	c. School of Nursing				
	d. Educational centers				
8.	**Lesson Plans**				
	a.				
	b.				
	c.				
	d.				
	e.				

Signature of Class Coordinator

Signature of the Principal

CLINICAL EVALUATION FORM FOR COMMUNITY HEALTH NURSING-I

Name: Ward:

Date: Total Marks: 25×4 = 100

KEY: 1. Unsatisfactory; 2. Satisfactory; 3. Good; 4. Very Good

Sl. No.		Very Good (4)	Good (3)	Fair (2)	Poor (1)	Not done (0)
1.	**Overall Evaluation**					
	Appearance					
	Uniform					
	Punctuality					
	Discipline					
	Team work					
	Attitude					
	Knowledge					
	Skill					
	Completing record book on time					
	Showing interest in learning					
2.	**Procedure Evaluation**					
	Participates in community survey					
	Does home visit					
	Assesses these environmental sanitation and nutrition					
	Application of standing orders					
3.	**Health Education**					
	Selects and prepares appropriate audio-visual aids					
	Uses audio-visual aids correctly					
	Timely gives health education as per need					
	• Individual					
	• Family					
	• Group					
	Respects the community practices					
	Follows bag technique					
	Assembles handles and replaces the articles properly					
	Involves in community health activities					
	Brings out innovative ideas to improve community development					

Contd...

Contd...

	Records and reports					
4.	**Growth and Development Including Nutrition**					
4.1	Assessment of growth and development					
	• Assessment of antenatal mother					
	• Assessment of newborn					
	• Assessment of infant					
	• Assessment of toddler					
	• Assessment of preschooler					
	• Assessment of schooler					
	• Assessment of adolescent					
	• Assessment of adult					
	• Assessment of elderly					
4.2	Assessment of nutritional status in various groups					
4.3	Diet planning for any age group					
	• Weaning diet					
	• Diet for pregnant mother					
	• Preparation of recipes					
	• Barley water					
	• Albumin water					
	• Lime whey					
	• Fluid diet					
	• Egg flip					
	• Dhal soup					
	• Vegetable soup					
	• Butter milk					
	• Light diet					
	• Toast					
	• Porridge					
	• Salads					
	• Jelly					
	• Arrow root					
	• Boiled water					
	• Custard egg					
	• Scrambled egg					
	• Steamed fish					
4.4	Visits					
	Postnatal ward, well baby clinic, creche/preschool food preparation and preservation center					

Remarks to Students

Positive Negative

1.

2.

3.

Total score for 25:

Signature of the Student *Signature of the Evaluator*

PRACTICAL EXAMINATION

Medical Surgical Nursing-I

Signature of Internal Examiner *Signature of External Examiner*

Date:

Repeat:

Signature of Internal Examiner *Signature of External Examiner*

Date:

Third Year

THIRD YEAR
HOURS OF INSTRUCTION

Theory: 300 hours **Clinical Experiences: 810 hours**

Sl. No.	Subjects	Theory (Hours)	Practical (Hours)	
1.	Medical Surgical Nursing (Adult Including Geriatrics)	120	270	
2.	Child Health Nursing	90	270	
3.	Mental Health Nursing	90	270	
4.	Nursing Research and Statistics	45	-	
5.	Library Work/Self-Study	-	-	50
6.	Co-curricular Activities	-	-	50
	Total	**345**	**810**	
	TOTAL HOURS: 1155			

Distribution of Subjects and Marks for Internal Assessment and University Examination

Sl. No.	Subjects	Hours	Internal assessment	External assessment	Total
1.	Medical Surgical Nursing	3	25	75	100
2.	Child Health Nursing	3	25	75	100
3.	Mental Health Nursing	3	25	75	100
4.	Nursing Research and Statistics	3	25	75	100
	Practical and Viva Voce				
1.	Medical Surgical Nursing-I		50	50	100
2.	Child Health Nursing		50	50	100
3.	Mental Health Nursing		50	50	100

Attendance of the student (%) :

Theory :

Clinical :

Signature of Class Coordinator *Signature of the Principal*

THIRD YEAR
MEDICAL SURGICAL NURSING-II

Sl. No.	Subjects	Class room		Clinical	
		Date	Signature	Date	Signature
1.	**Nursing Care of Adult Patient with ENT Disorders**				
	Examination of ear, nose and throat				
	History taking in ENT				
	Assisting with diagnostic procedures				
	• Speech test				
	• Tuning fork: Rinne and Weber test				
	• Finger friction test				
	• Audiometric test				
	• Tympanometry				
	• Throat swab culture				
	• Caloric test				
	Installation of drops				
	Application of ointments				
	Perform/assist irrigations				
	Assist in removal of foreign bodies				
	Emergency management in ENT conditions				
	Preparing and assisting in anterior/posterior nasal packing				
	Ear packing and syringing				
	Application of ear bandage				
	Tracheostomy care				
	Pre- and postoperative care of ENT surgeries				
	Teach patients and families				
	Sputum culture				
	Throat swab culture				
	Rhinoscopy				
	Nasopharyngoscopy				
	Identification of ENT disorders				
	Documentation of ENT procedures				
2.	**Nursing Care of Adult Patient with Eye Disorders**				
	Examination of eye				
	History taking in eye conditions				
	Assist in diagnostic procedures				
	• Fundoscopy				
	• Retinoscopy				
	• Ophthalmoscopy				
	• Refraction test				
	• Visual acuity				

Contd...

Contd...

	• Tonometry				
	• Syringing				
	Perform/assist in irrigation				
	Application of ointments				
	Perform/assist irrigations				
	Assist in removal of foreign bodies				
	Application of eye bandage				
	Pre- and postoperative care of eye surgeries				
	Assist in cataract surgery				
	Assist in minor ophthalmic surgeries				
	Teach patients and families				
	Emergency management in ophthalmic conditions				
	Identification of eye disorders				
	Documentation of ophthalmic procedures				
3.	**Nursing Care of Adult Patient with Neurological Disorders**				
	Neurological examination and History taking				
	Assist in diagnostic procedures				
	• Glasgow come scale				
	• Electroencephalogram (EEG)				
	• CT Scan				
	• Electromyography (EMG)				
	• Magnetic resonance imaging (MRI)				
	• Positron emission tomography (PET)				
	• Nerve conduction velocity (NCV)				
	• Electromyelography				
	• Evoked potentials				
	• Neurosonography				
	• Cerebral angiography				
	• Telemetry				
	• Lumbar puncture				
	Therapeutic procedure				
	• ICP monitoring				
	• Cervical traction				
	• Log rolling				
	Care of patient with				
	• Head injury				
	• Spinal cord injury				
	• Cerebrovascular accident				
	• Neurological emergencies				
	Pre- and postoperative care of neurological surgeries				
	Teach patients and families				
	Participate in rehabilitation program				

Contd...

Contd...

	Identification of neurological disorders				
	Documentation of neurological procedures				
4.	**Nursing Care of Adult Patient with Gynecological Disorders**				
	Gynecological examination and History taking				
	Assist in diagnostic procedures				
	• Self-breast examination (SBE)				
	• PAP smear				
	• Colposcopy				
	• Radiological testing: ultrasound				
	• Hysterosalpingography				
	• Hysteroscopy				
	• Loop electrical excision procedure (LEEP)				
	• Mammography				
	• Hormone imbalance testing				
	• Cystoscopy				
	• Biopsy: cervical and endometrial				
	Assist in therapeutic examination				
	• Copper-T insertion				
	• Dilation and curettage procedure				
	Assist in gynecological surgeries				
	Pre- and postoperative care of gynecological surgeries				
	Teach patients and families				
	Identification of gynecological disorders				
	Documentation of gynecological procedures				
5.	**Nursing Care of Adult Patient with Burns**				
	Burns assessment				
	Calculation of percentage and degree of burns				
	Calculation of fluid and electrolyte therapy				
	• Assess				
	• Calculate				
	• Replace				
	Record intake output chart				
	Promoting gas exchange and airway management				
	Restoring fluid & electrolytes				
	Pain management				
	Care of burn wounds				
	Bathing				
	Burns dressing				
	Perform active and passive exercises				
	Practice medical and surgical asepsis				
	Assist in reconstruction surgeries				
	Teach patients and families				

Contd...

Contd...

	Participate in rehabilitation program				
	Documentation of procedures in burns				
6.	**Nursing Care of Adult Patient with Cancer**				
	History taking and physical examination				
	Assessment of warning signals				
	TNM classifications				
	Self-breast examination				
	Assist in diagnostic procedures				
	• Biopsy				
	• Pap smear				
	• Bone marrow aspiration				
	• Mammography				
	• Endoscopic procedures				
	• Tumor markers				
	Assist in therapeutic procedures				
	Participate in various modalities of treatment				
	• Chemotherapy				
	• Radiotherapy				
	• Pain management				
	• Stoma therapy				
	• Hormonal therapy				
	• Immune therapy				
	• Gene therapy				
	• Alternative therapy				
	• Adjuvant therapy				
	Surgical interventions of cancer				
	Pre- and postoperative care				
	Pain management				
	Participate in palliative care				
	Counsel and teach patients and families				
	Participate in rehabilitation program				
	Palliative care				
	Stem cell transplantation				
	Genetic counseling				
	Promoting home and community based care				
	Documentation in oncology procedures				
7.	**Nursing Care of Adult Patient in Intensive Care Unit**				
	Assessment and history taking in ICU				
	Monitoring of patients in ICU				
	Maintain ICU flowchart				
	Care of patients in ventilator				
	Perform endotracheal suction				

Contd...

Contd...

	Demonstrate uses of				
	• Ventilator				
	• Cardiac monitors				
	• Infusion pumps				
	• ABG machine				
	• Pulse oximeter				
	• Defibrillator				
	Collect specimen and interpret ABG analysis				
	Assist with ICU procedures:				
	• CVP line				
	• Arterial line				
	• Central line				
	• Endotracheal tube				
	• Tracheostomy tube				
	• Chest tube				
	• Pace maker				
	• Bag mask ventilation				
	Assist and perform advanced cardiovascular resuscitation				
	Preparation of emergency trolley—Crash cart				
	Administration of drugs				
	• Infusion pump				
	• Epidural				
	• Intrathecal				
	• Total parenteral nutrition (TPN)				
	Physiotherapy—chest physio				
	Perform active and passive exercises				
	Counsel the patient and family in dealing with grieving and bereavement				
	Documentation in ICU procedures				
8.	**Nursing Care of Adult Patient in Emergency and Disaster Situation**				
	Emergency assessments				
	Practice triage				
	Code blue/green				
	Assist casualities				
	• Assessment				
	• Examination				
	• Investigation				
	• Implementation of care				
	Assist in legal practices/procedures during emergencies				
	Standing orders/protocols				
	Maintenance of recording in emergency situation				
	Counselling of family members during grief and bereavement				
	Documentation in emergency care				

Nursing Care Plan

Sl. No.	Care plan	Date	Signature
1.			
2.			
3.			
4.			
5.			

Case Studies

Sl. No.		Date	Signature
1.			
2.			
3.			
4.			

Case Presentation / Ward Teaching

Sl. No.		Date	Signature
1.			
2.			
3.			
4.			

Health Teaching

Sl. No.	Topic	Focused group	AV-Aids	Method	Date	Signature
1.						
2.						
3.						
4.						
5.						

Signature of Class Coordinator

Signature of the Principal

THIRD YEAR
CHILD HEALTH NURSING

Sl. No.	*Subjects*	*Classroom*		*Clinical*	
		Date	*Signature*	*Date*	*Signature*
1.	**Nursing Care of Children with Medical Disorders**				
	Admission procedure				
	Pediatric history				
	Physical examination				
	Administration of medication				
	• Oral				
	• Intramuscular				
	• Intravenous				
	• Suppositories				
	• Instillation of medications in eye, nose and ear				
	Calculation of fluid				
	Drug calculations				
	Prepare different strengths of IV Fluids				
	Restraints				
	• Elbow restraints				
	• Mummy restraints				
	• Jacket restraints				
	• Clove hitch restraints				
	• Mitten restraints				
	• Restraining limbs				
	• Hip spica				
	Oxygen therapy				
	Nasal catheter				
	Nasal cannula				
	• Mask: venturi				
	• Oxyhood				
	• Tent				
	• Baby bath				
	Feeding children by				
	• Formula preparation				
	• Katori and spoon				
	• Nasogastric tube feeding				
	• Breastfeeding				
	• Cleaning and sterilization of feeding instruments				
	Specimen collection				
	• Urine: culture and sensitivity				
	• Stool				
	• Blood specimen				

Contd...

Contd...

	• Sputum				
	• Throat swab				
	• Skin scraping				
	Assist with common diagnostic procedures				
	Assist with common therapeutic procedures				
	Teach mothers/parents				
	• Malnutrition				
	• Oral rehydration therapy				
	• Feeding and weaning				
	• Immunization schedule				
	• Play therapy				
	• Specific disease conditions				
2.	**Nursing Care of Children with Surgical Disorders**				
	Calculate and prepare and administer IV fluids				
	Bowel wash				
	Care of ostomies and irrigation:				
	• Colostomy				
	• Uretostomy				
	• Gastrostomy				
	• Entrostomy				
	Urinary catheterization and drainage				
	Male				
	Female				
	Feeding				
	• Nasogastric				
	• Gastrostomy				
	• Jejunostomy				
	• Feeding child with cleft lip and cleft palate				
	Surgical care				
	• Preoperative care				
	• Postoperative care				
	• Surgical wounds				
	• Surgical dressing				
	• Suture removal				
3.	**Perform Assessment of Children: Health, Developmental and Anthropometric**				
	Health assessment				
	Anthropometric measurements				
	• Height				
	• Weight				
	• Head circumferences				
	• Chest circumferences				
	• Mid-arm circumferences				

Contd...

Contd...

	Vital signs				
	• Temperature				
	– Oral				
	– Auxilla				
	– Rectal				
	• Pulse				
	• Respiration				
	• Blood pressure				
	Developmental mile stones				
	• 0–1 years				
	• 1–3 years				
	• 3–6 years				
	• 6–12 years				
	Immunization				
	• Oral				
	• Subcutaneous				
	• Intravenous				
	• Intramuscular				
	• Intradermal				
4.	**Nursing Care to Critically Ill Children**				
	Preparation of intensive care unit				
	Preparing emergency trolley				
	Care of child on mechanical ventilator				
	Endotracheal suctioning				
	Administering medicines through syringe/infusion pump				
	Assist in phototherapy				
	Total parenteral nutrition				
	Cardiopulmonary resuscitation				
	• Two finger technique				
	• Thumb technique				
	Monitoring the baby				
	Monitoring the child with pulse oximeter				
	Chest physiotherapy				
5.	**Neonatal Care**				
	Newborn assessment				
	Check and recording APGAR				
	Neonatal resuscitation (TCAB)				
	Care of new bone with following conditions:				
	• High-risk newborn				
	• Low-birth weight baby				
	• Preterm baby				
	• Small for date				

Contd...

Contd...

	• Congenital anomalies				
	• Photo-therapy				
	• Warmer				
	• Incubator				
	• Bilibanket/bilitherapy				
6.	**Pediatric Emergencies**				
	Head injury				
	Asphyxia				
	Hemolytic disorders				
	Convulsions				
	Accidents				
7.	**Assist in Therapeutic Procedure**				
	Lumbar puncture				
	Exchange transfusion				
	Blood transfusion				
8.	**Health Education/Teaching to Parents**				
	Supplementary foods				
	Special diet				
	Weaning				
	Hygiene				
	Immunization				
	Prevention of accidents				
	Developmental milestones				

Nursing Care Plan (Medical)

Sl. No.	*Care plan*	*Date*	*Signature*
1.			
2.			
3.			
4.			
5.			

Nursing Care Plan (Surgical)

Sl. No.	*Care plan*	*Date*	*Signature*
1.			
2.			
3.			
4.			
5.			

Case Studies

Sl. No.		Date	Signature
1.			
2.			
3.			
4.			

Case Presentation

Sl. No.		Date	Signature
1.			
2.			
3.			
4.			

Health Teaching

Sl. No.	Topic	Focused group	AV-Aids	Method	Date	Signature
1.						
2.						
3.						
4.						
5.						

Signature of Class Coordinator

Signature of the Principal

THIRD YEAR
MENTAL HEALTH NURSING

Sl. No.	Subjects	Classroom		Clinical	
		Date	Signature	Date	Signature
1.	**Assessment of Patients with Mental Health Problems**				
	History taking				
	Perform mental status examination				
	Mini mental status examination				
	Neurological examination				
	Psychological testing				
	Psychometric assessment				
	Physical investigation:				
	• CT Scan				
	• MRI				
	• EEG				
2.	**Psychiatric Admission and Discharge**				
	Voluntary admission				
	Involuntary admission				
	Emergency admission				
	Reception order				
	Temporary admission				
	Admission of criminal lunatics				
	Discharge of mentally ill clients				
3.	**Assist in Therapeutic Modalities**				
	Physical therapy				
	• Electroconvulsive therapy				
	• Care before ECT				
	• Care during ECT				
	• Care after ECT				
	Psychotherapies				
	• Behavior therapy				
	• Milieu therapy				
	• Aversion therapy				
	• Group therapy				
	• Hypnosis				
	• Psychoanalysis				
	• Family therapy				

Contd...

Contd...

	• Diversion therapy				
	• Individual psychotherapy				
	• Music therapy				
	• Dance therapy				
	• Recreation therapy				
	• Play therapy				
	• Occupational therapy				
	Psychopharmacological therapy				
	Narcoanalysis				
	Lithium therapy				
	Disulfiram therapy				
4.	**Assessment of Children with Various Mental Health Problems**				
	History taking				
	Assist in psychometric assessment				
	Observe and assist in various therapies				
	Care of child with				
	• Mental retardation				
	• Conduct disorders				
	Teach family and significant others				
5.	**Maintain Therapeutic Communication**				
6.	**Process Recording**				
7.	**Prepare Patients for Activities of Daily Living**				
8.	**Administration of Psychiatric Medications**				
9.	**Community Mental Health Services:**				
	Conduct case work				
	Identify individuals with mental health problems				
	Levels of preventions				
	Assist in mental health camps and clinics				
	Rehabilitation services				
	Participate in community mental health services				
	Counsel and teach family members, patients and community members				
10.	**Nursing care of clients with**				
	Schizophrenia				
	Mood disorders				
	Organic brain disorders				
	Psychiatric emergencies				
	Neurotic disorders				
	Substance abuse				

Contd...

Contd...

11.	**Observational visits**				
	Community mental health center				
	De-addiction center				
	Halfway home				
	Old age home				
	Rehabilitation center				
	School mental health services				

Nursing Care Plan

Sl. No.	*Care plan*	*Date*	*Signature*
1.			
2.			
3.			
4.			
5.			

Case Studies

Sl. No.		*Date*	*Signature*
1.			
2.			
3.			
4.			

Case Presentation/Ward Teaching

Sl. No.		*Date*	*Signature*
1.			
2.			
3.			
4.			

Process Recording

Sl. No.	*Name of the client*	*Diagnosis*	*Duration*	*Date of submission*	*Signature*
1.					
2.					
3.					
4.					
5.					

Mental Status Examination

Sl. No.	Name of the client	Diagnosis	Date of MSE	Date of submission	Signature
1.					
2.					
3.					
4.					
5.					

Health Teaching

Sl. No.	Topic	Focused group	AV-Aids	Method	Date	Signature
1.						
2.						
3.						
4.						
5.						

Signature of Class Coordinator *Signature of the Principal*

THIRD YEAR PRACTICAL EXAMINATION

Medical Surgical Nursing

Signature of Internal Examiner

Date:

Signature of External Examiner

Date:

Supplementary:

Signature of Internal Examiner:

Date:

Signature of External Examiner

Date:

Child Health Nursing

Signature of Internal Examiner:

Date:

Signature of External Examiner

Date:

Supplementary:

Signature of Internal Examiner:

Date:

Signature of External Examiner

Mental Health Nursing

Signature of Internal Examiner:

Date:

Signature of External Examiner

Date:

Supplementary:

Signature of Internal Examiner:

Date:

Signature of External Examiner

CLINICAL EVALUATION FORM FOR CHILD HEALTH NURSING

Name: Ward:

Area of Clinical Experience:

Date: From: To:

Sl. No.		*V. Good (4)*	*Good (3)*	*Fair (2)*	*Poor (1)*	*Not done (0)*
1.	**Professional Attitudes**					
	Demonstrate leadership abilities					
	Punctual in reporting					
	Establishing good rapport with staff and other students					
	Dependable and trustworthy					
	Demonstrates a good sense ethics in behavior					
	Works independently					
	Accepts constructive criticism					
2.	**Professional Competence**					
	Identifies and collects various source of data from client and family					
	Performs physical and mental status examination of the client					
	Collects other patient information					
	Analysis all the data collected					
	Accurately interprets and synthesis the information					
	Formulation of nursing diagnosis					
3.	**Planning**					
	Prioritize the problem and needs					
	Plans the appropriate nursing interventions					
	Involves the child and family in the planning					
4.	**Implementation/Professional Skills**					
	Implements nursing care applying the principles of child and family care					
	Establishes good rapport with child and family					
	Utilizes available resources in carrying out nursing care					
	Educates the child and family in accordance with their learning needs					
5.	**Evaluation**					
	Evaluates the nursing care rendered					
	Revises the nursing care plan when needed					
6.	**Documentation**					
	Records and reports promptly					
	Acts as a resource person in clinical settings					

Marks Obtained:

Key		Marks
1. Consistent practice	:	04
2. Practice regularly with few errors	:	03
3. Practice sometimes with many errors	:	02
4. Practice rarely	:	01
5. Never practice	:	00

Signature of the Student

Date:

Comments:

Signature of the Supervisor

Date:

Comments:

Fourth Year

FOURTH YEAR
HOURS OF INSTRUCTION

Theory: 315 hours **Clinical Experiences: 780 hours**

Sl. No.	*Subjects*	*Theory (Hours)*	*Practical (Hours)*
1.	Midwifery and Obstetrical Nursing	90	600
2.	Community Health Nursing	90	135
3.	Management of Nursing Services and Education	60 + 30	
	Total	**270**	**735**
	TOTAL HOURS: 1005		

Distribution of Subjects and Marks for Internal Assessment and University Examination

Sl. No.	*Subjects*	*Hours*	*Internal assessment*	*External assessment*	*Total*
1.	Midwifery and Obstetrical Nursing	3	25	75	100
2.	Community Health Nursing-II	3	25	75	100
3.	Management of Nursing Service and Education	3	25	75	100
	Practical and Viva Voce				
1.	Midwifery and Obstetrical Nursing		50	50	100
2.	Community Health Nursing		50	50	100

Attendance of the student (%) :

Theory :

Clinical :

Signature of Class Coordinator *Signature of the Principal*

FOURTH YEAR
MIDWIFERY AND OBSTETRICAL NURSING (NORMAL)

Sl. No.	Subjects	Classroom		Clinical	
		Date	Signature	Date	Signature
1.	**Assessment of Pregnant Women**				
	Antenatal history taking				
	Physical examination				
	Calculating				
	• **Expected date of delivery (EDD)**				
	• **Obstetrical score**				
	• **Gestational weeks**				
	Recording of				
	• Vital signs				
	• Weight				
	• Blood pressure				
	• Hemoglobin				
	• Urine: sugar and albumin				
	• Urine pregnancy test				
	Antenatal examination				
	• Abdomen: inspection, palpation and auscultation				
	• Breast examination				
	• Estimation of gestational age				
	• Measuring fundal height				
	Immunization				
	Assessment of risk status				
	Teaching antenatal mothers				
	Maintenance of antenatal records				
	Antenatal exercise				
2.	**Assessment of Women in Labor**				
	Preparation for labor				
	Assist in setting labor room				
	Setting up of newborn resuscitation unit				
	Assessment of women in labor				
	Per vaginal examination (PV)				
	Maintenance of partograph				
	Bishops score				
	Monitoring and caring of women in labor				
	Perineal preparation of mother for labor				
	Monitoring and recording uterine contraction and relaxation chart				
	Monitoring and recording of FSH				
	Administer soap and water enema				
	Maintain labor progress chart				

Contd...

Contd...

	Monitoring and recording of cervical dilatation and fetal descent				
	Conducting normal deliveries				
	Newborn assessment				
	Immediate care of newborn				
	• Cord care				
	• Warming				
	• Bathing				
	• Rooming in				
	• Assistance in feeding				
	• Immunization				
	Resuscitation of newborn				
	Episiotomy and suturing				
	Maintain records and reports				
	Arrange and assist in MTP procedures				
	Arrange and assist in other surgical procedures				
	Cesarean section: care of mother and baby				
3.	**Providing Nursing Care to Postnatal Mother**				
	Preparing postnatal unit				
	Postnatal assessment and examination of mother				
	Postnatal assessment and examination of baby				
	Perineal care				
	Assist in breastfeeding				
	Baby bath				
	Immunization to baby				
	Lactation management				
	Registration of birth				
	Teaching postnatal exercises				
	Teaching mother craft				
	Teaching mother regarding diet				
	Maintenance of records and reports				
	Postnatal exercises				
	Identifying the postnatal complications				
4.	**Nursing Care Newborn at Risk**				
	Newborn assessment				
	Feeding of at risk neonates				
	• Katori spoon				
	• Paladin				
	• Tube feeding				
	• Total parental nutrition (TPN)				
	Thermal management of neonates				
	• Kangaroo mother care				
	• Incubator care				

Contd...

Contd...

	Monitoring and care of neonates				
	Administering medications				
	Intravenous therapy				
	Assisting with diagnostic procedures				
	• Ventilator care				
	• Phototherapy				
	Infection control protocols in the nursery				
	Teaching and counseling of parents				
	Maintenance of records				
5.	**Family Welfare Services**				
	Counseling techniques				
	Insertion of IUD				
	Teaching on use of family planning methods				
	Arrange for and assist with family planning operations				
	Maintenance of records and reports				
	Requirements				
	Antenatal examination-30				
	Conducting normal deliveries-20				
	Vaginal examination-5				
	Episiotomy and suturing-5				
	Neonatal resuscitation-5				
6.	**Observational visits**				
	Postpartum center				
	Family planning clinic/family welfare center				
	Under five clinic				
	MCH clinic				
	Voluntary health agencies				

Nursing Care Plan

Sl. No.	*Care plan*	*Date*	*Signature*
1.			
2.			
3.			
4.			
5.			

Case Studies

Sl. No.		*Date*	*Signature*
1.			
2.			
3.			
4.			

Case Presentation / Ward Teaching

Sl. No.		Date	Signature
1.			
2.			
3.			
4.			

Health Teaching

Sl. No.	Topic	Focused group	AV-Aids	Method	Date	Signature
1.						
2.						
3.						
4.						
5.						

Signature of Class Coordinator

Signature of the Principal

FOURTH YEAR
MIDWIFERY AND OBSTETRICAL NURSING (ABNORMAL)

		OBG-lab		*Clinical*	
Sl. No.	***Subjects***	***Date***	***Signature***	***Date***	***Signature***
1.	**Nursing Care Antenatal Mother**				
	Setting up of antenatal clinic				
	Setup of obstetric ICU				
	Setup of eclampsia unit				
	Assessment of high-risk pregnancies				
	Care of high-risk antenatal women				
	• Pre-eclampsia				
	• Eclampsia				
	• Placenta previa				
	• Abruptio placenta				
	• Gestational diabetes				
	• Cardiac disease				
	• Rh-compactability				
	• Preterm labor				
	• Anemia				
	Care of pregnant women with gynecological problems				
	Care of mother with HIV/AIDS				
	Documentation: recording and reporting				
2.	**Nursing Care in Labor Room**				
	Assist in setting labor room				
	Assessment of women in labor				
	Per vaginal examination				
	Maintenance of partograph				
	Monitoring and caring of women in labor				
	Perineal preparation of mother for labor				
	Monitoring and recording uterine contraction and relaxation chart				
	Monitoring and recording of FSH				
	Administer soap and water enema				
	Maintain labor progress chart				
	Monitoring and recording of cervical dilatation and fetal descent				
	Conducting normal deliveries				
	Documentation				
3.	**Management of Abnormal Labor**				
	Obstructed labor				
	Induction of labor				
	Assist in deliveries with abnormal presentation				
	• Forceps delivery				
	• Vacuum delivery				

Contd...

Contd...

	• Breech delivery				
	• Face and brow				
	• Multifetal delivery				
	• Cesarean section				
	Assist in obstetrical emergencies				
	• Rupture of uterus				
	• Placenta previa				
	• Hemorrhage and shock				
	• Cord prolapsed				
	• Abruptio placenta				
	Arranging and assisting in various surgical procedures				
	• Episiotomy				
	• Hysterectomy				
	• Manual removal of placenta				
	• Cesarean section				
	• Dilatation and curettage (D & E)				
	• Dilatation and evacuation (D & E)				
	• Version				
	• Laparoscopy				
4.	**Nursing Management of Postnatal Mother**				
	Puerperal care				
	Perineal care				
	Perineal light				
	Care of high-risk postnatal mothers				
	• Postpartum hemorrhage				
	• Infection				
	• Breast disorders				
	• Sub-involution				
	Mental disorders				
	• Postpartum depression				
	• Postpartum blue				
	• Postpartum psychosis				
5.	**Nursing Management of High-risk Newborn**				
	Assessment of preterm baby				
	Care of high-risk neonates				
	• Preterm baby				
	• Low-birth weight baby				
	• Asphysia				
	Nursing care high-risk newborn				
	• Phototherapy				
	• Radiant warmer				
	• Ventilator care				
	• Incubator care				

Contd...

Contd...

	Administration of medication				
	Maintenance of neonatal records				
	Teaching the parents of high-risk neonates				
	NICU protocols				
	Newborn resuscitation				
6.	**Family Welfare and Planning Services**				
	Motivation of planned parenthood				
	Arrange and assist in copper-T insertion				
	Assist in MTP				
	Assist in tubectomy				
	Assist in vasectomy				
	Arrange counseling services: infertility clinic				
	Maintain records and reports				
7.	**Observational visits**				
	Postpartum center				
	Family planning clinic/family welfare center				
	Under five clinic				
	MCH clinic				
	Voluntary health agencies				
8.	**Requirements**				
	Witness abnormal deliveries-10				
	Assist in abnormal deliveries-5				
	Motivation of parenthood-2				
	Attend ANC and PNC clinic-1 week				
	Provide care to high-risk antenatal mothers-5				
	Provide care to high-risk neonates-5				
	Provide care to high-risk postnatal mothers-5				
	Witness cesarean section-5				

Antenatal High-risk Nursing Care Plan/Case Study

Sl. No.	*Care plan*	*Date*	*Signature*
1.			
2.			
3.			
4.			
5.			

Postnatal High-risk Nursing Care Plan/Case Study

Sl. No.		*Date*	*Signature*
1.			
2.			
3.			
4.			

Neonatal High-risk Nursing Care Plan / Case Study

Sl. No.		*Date*	*Signature*
1.			
2.			
3.			
4.			

Health Teaching

Sl. No.	*Topic*	*Focused group*	*AV-Aids*	*Method*	*Date*	*Signature*
1.						
2.						
3.						
4.						
5.						

Completion of Internship—5 Weeks

Sl. No.	*Internship -obstetrical nursing-labor ward/ ANC/NICU/antenatal/Postnatal ward*	*Duration*	*Date*	*Signature*
1.	Comprehensive care of antenatal mother	1 week		
2.	Comprehensive care of mother in labor/OT	2 weeks		
3.	Comprehensive care of postnatal mother	1 week		
4.	Comprehensive care of high-risk newborn	1 week		
5.	Completion of casebook recordings			

Signature of Class Coordinator *Signature of the Principal*

FOURTH YEAR
COMMUNITY HEALTH NURSING-II

Sl. No.	Subjects	Community lab		Clinical	
		Date	Signature	Date	Signature
1.	**Community Health Survey**				
2.	**Preparing Map of Community Area**				
3.	**Community Health Process**				
	• Assessment				
	• Community diagnosis				
	• Planning				
	• Implementation				
	• Evaluation				
4.	**Family Health Assessment**				
5.	**Family Care: Home Adaptation of Common Procedures**				
	• Vital signs				
	• Dressing				
	• Baby bath				
	• Urine test: sugar and albumin				
	Demonstration of care				
	• Care of fever patient				
	• Oral rehydration therapy				
	Nutritional assessment				
6.	**Home Visit**				
7.	**Bag Technique**				
8.	**Immunization/Vaccination**				
9.	**Organize and Conduct Clinics**				
	• Antenatal				
	• Postnatal				
	• Well baby clinic				
	• MCH clinic				
	• Family planning clinic				
	• Under five clinic				
	• School health clinic				
	• Geriatric clinic				
	• Health camps				
10.	**Screen, Manage and Referrals for**				
	• High-risk mother				
	• High-risk neonates				
	• Accidents				
	• Emergencies				
	• Physical and mental illness				
	• Disabilities				

Contd...

Contd...

11.	**Midwifery and Child Health Services**				
	Antenatal assessment				
	Antenatal examination				
	Abdominal examination				
	Measuring fundal height				
	Abdominal palpation				
	Checking and recording FSH				
	Record uterine contraction and dilatation				
	Antenatal care and advice				
	Conducting deliveries at center				
	Conducting deliveries at home				
	Episiotomy and suturing				
	Neonatal resuscitation				
	Immediate newborn care				
	• Oral suctioning				
	• Warming				
	• Rooming in				
	• Assist in breastfeeding				
	• Cord care				
	• Immunization				
	Postnatal care				
	• Postnatal exercises				
	• Postnatal advice				
12.	**Family Planning and Family Welfare Services**				
	Oral contraceptives				
	Injectable contraceptives				
	Condoms—male and female				
	Assisting in copper-T insertion				
	Assisting in permanent methods of sterilization				
	• Tubectomy				
	• Vasectomy				
	Assisting in MTP/abortion				
13.	**Vital Statistics**				
	Assisting and collecting vital statistics				
	• Birth and death registers				
	• Censes				
14.	**School Health Services**				
	School health assessment				
	Identification of high-risk individuals				
	Manage minor illnesses				
	Referrals for major illness				

Contd...

Contd...

15.	**Conducting and Teaching of Individual, Family and Community Regarding**				
	HIV/AIDS				
	Tuberculosis				
	Leprosy				
	Diabetes				
	Hypertension				
	Old age problems				
	Mental health problems				
	Physically challenged children				
	Adolescent				
16.	**Training and Supervision of Health Workers**				
17.	**Health Education**				
	• Individual				
	• Family				
	• Group				
	• Community/mass				
18.	**Assist and Maintain Various Records and Reports**				
	ANC register				
	Eligible couple register				
	Immunization register				
	Family planning register				
	Stock register				
	Family folder				
	Birth and death register				
	Writing community reports				
	Epidemic reports				
	Reports on National Health Program				
	Maintain individual and family records				
	Maintain administrative records				
19.	**Community Projects**				
20.	**Observational Visits**				
	School				
	Industry				
	Community Mental Health Center				
	National Family Planning Association of India				
	National Institute of Tuberculosis				
	Red cross/ WHO / UNICEF				
	Professional bodies: TNAI / INC / State Nursing Council				
	Isolation hospital				
	Leprosy sanatoriums				

Community Survey Report

Sl. No.	Area of survey	Type of survey	Duration of survey	Date of submission	Signature
1.					
2.					
3.					
4.					
5.					

Family Case Studies

Sl. No.	Name of the family	Identified health problems	Duration of study	Signature
1.				
2.				
3.				
4.				

Health Teaching

Sl. No.	Topic	Focused group	AV-Aids	Method	Date	Signature
1.						
2.						
3.						
4.						
5.						

Project Report

Sl. No.	Topic of project	Type Ist /group	Duration of project	Date of submission	Signature
1.					
2.					
3.					
4.					

Completion of Internship—9 Weeks

Sl. No.	Areas	Internship–Community Health Nursing-II	Duration	Date	Signature
1.	Urban	• Comprehensive care of two individual, family and community • Community Survey Report-1 • Family Care Study-1	5 weeks		
2.	Rural	Comprehensive care of two individual, family and community	4 weeks		
3.		Community Survey Report-1			
4.		Family Care Study-1			
5.		Case Book Recording			

Signature of Class Coordinator

Signature of the Principal

CLINICAL EVALUATION FORM FOR COMMUNITY HEALTH NURSING – II

Name of the Student: Duration:

Group and Class: Evaluator:

Date of Submission:

Sl. No.		*Good (3)*	*Fair (2)*	*Poor (1)*	*Not done (0)*
1.	**General**				
	Orientation to all allotted community area, population, etc.				
	Knows the responsibilities of community health nursing				
	Able to assess the community and family				
	Respects the belief and culture of the people				
	Knows to utilize the community resources				
	Identifies the risk factors and try to solve them				
	Compares the primary health care and national health programmers within the community				
2.	**Primary Health Centers (PHC)**				
	Learns the organization set up and function of PHC				
	Participate as a health team member in providing community health nursing services				
	Participate in training programs conducted by PHCs				
3.	Keeps the community health bag neat, clean and aseptic				
	Handles the bag appropriately and scientifically				
	Follows safe disposal method				
	Does home vIsIt				
	Provided home care as per the need				
	Involves members in community activities				
	Gives appropriate, planned health teaching				
	Brings changes in health practices for example: Diet, hygiene, exercise, etc.				
	Submits the community case study and record book on time				
	Prepared relevant statistics for the community area				
4.	**Maintains the Following Records Appropriately**				
	Family folder				
	Obstetrical record (antenatal to family planning)				
	Pediatric record (newborn and under five)				
	Chronic illness record				
	School health record				

Remarks of Students

Positive
1.
2

Negative
1.

Signature of the Student *Signature of the Supervisor*

NURSING ADMINISTRATION

Sl. No.	*Topic*	*Date of instruction*	*Signature*
1.	**Supervision**		
	Students		
	Staffs		
	Ward aids		
2.	**Preparation of Duty Roster**		
	Preparation of work assignments		
	Students		
	Staff		
	Ward aids		
3.	**Report**		
	a. Oral		
	• Morning		
	• Evening		
	• Night		
	b. Written		
	• Day		
	• Night		
4.	**Inventory**		
	Drugs		
	Articles		
5.	**Maintenance Census**		
6.	**Conduct Nursing Rounds**		
	Clinical teaching		
7.	**Preparation of Job Description for Different Categories**		
	Principal		
	Nursing Superintendent		
	Clinical Instructors		
	Ward Sister/Head Nurse		
	Staff Nurse		
	Ward Aids		
8.	**Preparation of Evaluation Tool to Assess the Patients Care**		
9.	**Educational Tour to Various Institution and Professional Bodies and Submit the Report**		

Signature of Class Coordinator *Signature of the Principal*

PRACTICAL EXAMINATION

1. Midwifery Including Maternity and Gynecological Nursing-II

Signature of Internal Examiner *Signature of External Examiner*

Date:

Repeat:

Signature of Internal Examiner *Signature of External Examiner*

Date:

2. Community Health Nursing- II

Signature of Internal Examiner *Signature of External Examiner*

Date:

Repeat:

Signature of Internal Examiner *Signature of External Examiner*

Date:

NURSING RESEARCH AND STATISTICS

Clinical Experiences
Practical: 45 hours

Instruction

Title of the study should decided after research proposal, project done can be individual can group decided based on institution policies.

Sl. No.	*Procedure of Research*	*Date*	*Signature of the Guide*
1.	Critique the Published Research Nursing Journal-2		
2.	Research Proposal-1 (Individual/Group)		
3.	Statement of Problem, Formation of Conceptual Framework		
4.	Review of Literature, Research Methodology		
5.	Tool Construction		
6.	Tool-Reliability, Validity		
7.	Pilot Study		
8.	Methods of Data Collection		
9.	Statistical Analysis		
10.	Analysis and Interpretation		
11.	Reporting, Findings and Recommendations		
12.	Summary, Conclusion		
13.	Bibliography, References, Activities to be Done		
14.	Informed Consent		
15.	Permission Letters to Conduct Research		
16.	Final Presentation of Research in the Class/Clinicals		

CLINICAL POSTING FOR THE BASIC BSc NURSING STUDENTS

Month	First Year	Second Year	Third Year	Fourth Year	Any Other
September					
October					
November					
December					
January					
February					
March					
April					
May					
June					
July					
August					

Signature of Class Coordinator

Signature of the Principal